HOW TO LOSE WEIGHT NATURALLY

(Lose it all)

Table of Contents

Introduction

Have you ever considered to yourself that you could physically appear a little better, if not a lot better, than you do when you look in the mirror? If this is the case, you are not alone in your thoughts!

Our appetite for fatty meals and lack of exercise is an increasing worry around the world, statistics show that our health is rapidly deteriorating. We used to be able to indulge because we worked hard in physically demanding jobs, especially heavy labor, which meant calories were burnt throughout the day as we worked ourselves to exhaustion from morning to night.

This is no longer the case. With the rising popularity of computers and video games, as well as children spending more and more time surfing endlessly on social networking groups rather than spending time outside, things are looking bleak not only for the current generation, but also for future generations who will be exposed to the same lifestyle that we all enjoy (and suffer through without truly knowing it.)

Unfortunately, the weight-loss industry is thriving at our expense, thanks to mass-marketing of worthless, instant-results fat-loss solutions. People invest tens of millions of dollars in this industry in the hopes of getting the outcomes promised. However, there are no such things as rapid results, and these diet fads do not work.

In life, just one thing works, and that is hard effort! But it's not nearly as difficult as you imagine. It's all about seeing through the hype and forcing yourself to accept reality as it is, then moving on with a positive attitude and effort.

Amazing results can be achieved with a basic diet and a little exercise! Most people give up when they don't see quick results, yet results take time to manifest because nothing is instantaneous. This is where willpower comes into play to keep you on course. You will succeed if you can keep focused on your objective of losing weight and getting in shape.

The steps that follow are designed to assist you in achieving your objectives. Keep your sights on the prize, stay concentrated, and maintain a positive mindset, and the pounds will melt away!

What quantity do you need?

How much food do you eat on a daily basis? How much calorie-dense or fatty food are you consuming without even realizing it? The easiest method to figure out where your eating habits are going awry is to start looking at the nutrition facts on the packaging of the foods you're consuming and keeping a daily track of them for approximately a week. You'll be able to see where you're going wrong and where you need to improve in order to attain the outcomes you want.

The unpleasant reality is that we are more concerned with our taste buds than with healthy nourishment. This is the cause of weight growth and, eventually, obesity. Worse, most individuals find fast food far more handy than spending time in the kitchen preparing a tasty meal. The desire for ease in today's society is a major contributor to the rising obesity figures.

This is why, as a first step, it's critical to keep track of the meals you're taking into your body so you can assess the regions that require the most attention. By keeping track of the nutritional content of the meals you eat, you'll be able to figure out what's causing you to gain weight. After that, you can start reducing your fat intake and replace fatty foods with slightly healthier options.

A pound of fat has 3500 calories therefore, you'd have to remove 500 calories from your diet per week to lose a pound of fat. If you consume around 3000 calories per day, you may lose weight by removing 500 calories from that total by replacing poor meals with better ones and/or adding activity to your regular routine. By removing those 500 bad calories, you've reduced your calorie intake to 2500, and on top of that, you've decided to exercise for a half hour or 45 minutes on the treadmill, bike, or elliptical. With just over an hour of exercising and a better dinner, you'll be down to 2000 calories for the day. That'll be 2 pounds off your physique by the end of the week... and you'll probably feel lot better both mentally and physically as a result.

Not only do you break a good sweat throughout your workout, but your heart and entire body also receive a good workout, which means you're on your way to a healthy lifestyle. As always, combining eating less or choosing healthier meals with a little exercise can yield some truly impressive results, giving you not only increased self-confidence but also a vote of confidence from your family and friends.

The worst thing you can do is go on a crash diet, which is a severe tactic that involves going on a hunger strike in the hopes of losing weight quickly! This will only end in disaster as you will suffer hunger pains, forcing your body to feast on your muscle tissue, and you will eventually go on a serious food binge.

The tried-and-true strategy of eating healthier foods and getting more activity into your day will always yield positive outcomes.

A Better Option

Once you've determined how many unneeded calories you consume on a daily basis, you'll need to select where in your diet to make changes so that healthier meals take precedence over fatty items.

If you contemplate the Big Mac from McDonald's, which contains not only a lot of calories but also a lot of unhealthy ingredients, you might want to consider downsizing to a hamburger, which, while still not a healthy food, is considerably lower in calories and easier on the health.

Take, for example, a Burger King flame-broiled Whopper, which is really larger than the Big Mac. A single cheese Whopper has over 750 calories and about 50 grams of fat. Simply reducing to a mayo-free junior-sized Whopper may save 480 calories and 36 grams of fat. By substituting a smaller piece of fries for the larger ones, you will avoid consuming a large number of calories. If you're still hungry, a bowl of grapes or an apple would be a better choice than a second burger.

Some fast-food businesses, such as KFC, have begun to provide healthier options, such as grilled chicken in addition to fried chicken. KFC's grilled chicken breast and drumstick with mashed potatoes and gravy has a calorie count of around 400 calories and a fat content of little over 12 grams. On the other hand, the extra crispy chicken breast, which some say tastes no better than conventional fried chicken, has roughly 500 calories and more than 30 grams of fat after sitting in the deep fryer for a longer period of time.

Try a thin-crust at Domino's with ham and pineapple instead of pepperoni if you need a quick fix but also something nice and find pizza to be a really gratifying convenience. You've just conserved approximately 200 calories from entering your body.

It's also important not to overlook the pleasure of satisfying thirst with a calorie-dense milkshake! It tastes fantastic, but happily, they come in a variety of sizes, so you may have your favorite milkshake while also opting for a smaller cup. A triple-thick strawberry shake in the king size, for example, contains nearly 1000 calories! A modest portion contains 420 calories. If you want to lose weight, skip the shake and order an orange juice instead!

Let's not forget about breakfast! People need a good meal in the early morning rush hour to re-energize and get their bearings for another long day at the workplace combined with a tedious drive back and forth. The popular Egg McMuffin is a popular breakfast item in the United States however, it has 300 calories. The English Muffin, on the other hand, is half the size. This is the point at which you decide whether or not to order the less-fattening option. Despite the fact that none of it is nutritious, even choosing to downsize your portion or order the healthier dish can make a significant difference in your weight loss efforts.

Fast food has a strong hold on the American psyche. Fast food entails not just food on the go, but also convenience, as it is far easier to go through the drive-thru than it is to rummage through the fridge and put together a nutritious dinner. So why go to the hassle of cooking your own food when fast food is so easy to come by and is available everywhere you go? Even if fast food is quick, one can still choose from a variety of healthier options on the menu. You can gradually choose healthier foods or vary up your normal choices, similar to how you can downsize quantities from large to tiny.

The nutritional value of every product is listed on the container, so it's always a good idea to consider what you're putting into your body. There's no excuse for blaming the fast-food business or anyone else for your unhealthy shape or inability to lose weight if you keep a close check on what you consume. Fast food is convenient, but you are solely responsible for what you eat and have a choice, which is why it is advisable to keep a tight eye on the foods you consume when beginning your journey to a better lifestyle.

Moreover, decreasing weight is merely the first step. After a while, if you don't maintain your new eating habits, you may gain weight again. Snacking on junk food is acceptable if done in moderation and in conjunction with a healthy diet. Satisfying a hunger isn't necessarily a negative thing, but sticking to a reasonably healthy diet and getting some exercise on a daily basis is critical to improving your shape and leading to a healthier body and lifestyle.

Reduce the Size of Your Meals

One of the most important aspects of losing weight is to divide meals into smaller amounts rather than eating large meals all at once. It's been established that restricting your meals not only cuts down on your caloric intake throughout the day, but it also helps to keep your metabolism in check. Consider eating 6-7 smaller meals throughout the day if you're used to eating 2-3 large meals per day.

People prefer to eat directly from the package rather than removing what they require and discarding the packet. Eating a mega-sized packet of potato chips is an illustration of this. Not only do you have no idea how much you're eating, but you're usually gratifying a hunger by eating more than you need until you're entirely pleased when you could alternatively pour a small portion into a bowl and add a piece of fruit to receive the exact amount of food you require.

Super-sized packs are more frequent now than they were previously. More foods are provided in restaurants with the option to super-size for a few more pennies, and more things are sold in bulk. Increased portion sizes are contributing to rising obesity rates. There is always a reason, yet individuals choose pleasure over all else, putting their health at risk. This is why restricting meals is a useful tool for breaking harmful behaviors. Making changes takes discipline, and there's no reason why individuals should feel obligated to eat until they're satisfied. Tiny quantities are good, and if you're still hungry, add a little more rather than filling your plate and trying to finish it all. Rather than sitting around feeling stuffed and removing your belt buckle, allowing some room for another modest meal a few hours later but still feeling well enough to do some exercise is a healthy balance that leads to better results. This helps you control your weight and it gradually starts to come down, which is a wonderful sensation that motivates you to work a little more as you gain confidence in your ability to control your own body rather than allowing your urges to rule you.

Are You Getting Enough Fiber?

What exactly is fiber, and why is it necessary in our diets? Fiber, simply said, helps to reduce the risk of a variety of serious illnesses and disorders, including diabetes, heart disease, diverticulitis, and even stroke. It also curbs your cravings for more food by assisting you in obtaining the satisfaction you require, ensuring that you do not require any additional food or as much food as you desire.

The average daily fiber consumption for men is 30 grams and for women it is 20 grams. Fruits and vegetables, as well as beans and whole grain breads, are excellent sources of fiber. Raisin Bran

Extra has roughly 7 grams of fiber, which is an excellent amount for morning cereals.

Rapidly boosting your fiber intake is never a good idea, so if your body is used to getting around 10-15 grams of fiber per day, don't start eating 30 grams right once. The body must adapt gradually, over the course of a month. There are plenty of fiber-rich meals to choose from, and you can aim to consume more of these instead of the ones that are lower in fiber.

As previously stated, juice products are far healthier than shakes. Natural fruits, such as oranges and apples, offer more fiber and less calories than juices. Bananas, grapes, and other fruits can be added to your breakfast. You can even include crackers, which are high in fiber.

Whole wheat breads, crackers, and some cereals

are high in fiber and provide an excellent start to

your day. You can also include beans in your

breakfast or lunch because they are high in fiber

and contain protein, which aids muscular growth.

Turn On the Treadmill

Few people like working out. It's like walking up a hill when you exercise and see results. It necessitates an effort, which most people dislike because effort equates to work. On the other hand, just like descending down the hill, it's simple to gain weight by doing nothing. Physical activity can be difficult for certain people due to hurting knees or back problems, for example. However, there are ways to incorporate some activity into your daily routine. Any little bit helps, whether it's to use an elliptical machine instead of running, or to use an exercise bike instead of bicycling over trails and rocky terrains, or to just pick up a tennis racquet and squeeze a little session into your evenings by hitting with your friends or family.

The Wii Fit, thanks to technology and video games, allows you to participate in exciting training routines in the comfort of your own living room while keeping track of your fitness level and calories expended.

Furthermore, there are activities such as tennis, boxing, and bowling that require real-motion movement, allowing you to get physically involved while also having fun.

If your goal is to lose a couple of pounds every week, it's improbable that you'll burn 500 or more calories in a single session if you're new to exercise. A person weighing 165 pounds or less is unlikely to burn 500 calories in just 30 minutes of football, tennis, or jogging. Cutting that many calories would necessitate a greater effort and a longer period of time. However, just as you may break up your meals throughout the day to achieve your goals, you can likewise divide up your exercise routines throughout the day to achieve your goals.

One of the best things about exercise, particularly cardio-type training, is that you can do it at different times of the day and still get the same results as if you did it all at once. If you regularly get up at 6:30 a.m. to get ready for work, try getting up even earlier at 6:00 a.m. and going for a 30-minute treadmill run before getting into the shower. Not only will you have had a fantastic workout, but you'll also be exceptionally fresh, alert, and inspired before going to work.

A 30-minute run can burn 400-500 calories at a moderate pace, depending on your level of fitness, but you can also perform a brisk stroll and burn 200 or more calories. After work, you can consider going for an evening stroll, cycling, or even playing a sport like soccer, basketball, or tennis...basically anything that will help you break a sweat and get your body moving.

During rainy days or the winter season, you might want to consider getting a gym membership and trying out the various cardio machines offered, such as the treadmill and exercise cycle, as well as the elliptical, stair climber, and rowing machine.

Everything there is meant to get your heart racing and help you work up a good sweat. You can always start slowly and gradually increase your speed over time. Never push yourself harder than your body can manage in the beginning. Over time, you will naturally improve, and your health will considerably improve as well.

Your Best Friend Is Water

According to study, you should drink at least 8 glasses of water every day, although the amount you need will vary depending on your weight. You would divide your weight by two, thus a man weighing 180 pounds would require 60 ounces of water each day.

So, why do experts advise us to drink plenty of water, and why is it considered so important to living a healthy lifestyle? To begin with, it helps to prevent dehydration and keeps the kidneys operating properly by assisting in the elimination of waste items, as well as increasing your metabolism, which aids in weight loss.

However, in addition to listening to what experts have to say, you should prioritize listening to your body. When you are thirsty, you will naturally drink water to quench your thirst. Depending on the type of work you do, you should aim to get into the habit of drinking water on a regular basis or, better yet, keeping a water bottle on hand, especially on extremely hot days when your body sweats and loses water, necessitating replenishment.

This is why water is so vital to human survival. Not only does it have no calories, but it is also the healthiest way to quench your thirst. You may want to gradually add water to all of your meals, eventually replacing fruit drinks and sodas with water, as this will help you reduce your caloric intake and you'll feel much better without the extra sugar in the other drinks.

Ready...Set...Go!

Everyone believes they know what they should do. They read the content, recognize that they must act and exert effort, but they rarely do so. It will be tough to begin on the road to a healthy life unless you discipline yourself to resist the temptation of eating unhealthy foods and drive yourself to eat healthy foods.

If you don't take that first step, no amount of reading or repeating "Yes, I can do it" would help you. It takes a lot of effort to get back on track, and it takes much more effort to stay on track. Because they are dissatisfied with their achievements, most people give up after a short period. You will attain your goal if you can commit, stay inspired, and continue to aim to eat good and exercise well. Whatever your aim is, whether it's to lose weight, boost your endurance, or improve your performance in a certain sport, all you have to do is put in the effort and put in the work.

Not only will you mentally acclimatize to your workout regimen over time, but you will also gain a great deal of discipline and self-confidence, as well as a natural good attitude, allowing you to effortlessly resist any form of temptation. Everybody has to get started someplace. Setting small goals rather than going all-out and aiming to lose 10 pounds on the treadmill in a week would do more harm than good. It's important to ease into the process, which means going for a quick walk to help your body adjust to the more strenuous runs you'll be doing in the coming weeks.

People make the mistake of going all out when they first start out, which leads to injury and them deciding that training is too difficult and taxing. Set a timetable like before, and if you're having trouble coming up with one, talk to a personal trainer about what could work best for you. You don't have to make the procedure so complicated. If you want to lose weight, all you need is a brief daily window dedicated to exercise and a close eye on what you put into your body.

Simply be self-assured and work toward your objectives. Maintain a good attitude and you will achieve your goals. Perhaps now is a wonderful time to start making that plan and putting it into

action so you can start living the extremely healthy

lifestyle you deserve

www.ingramcontent.com/pod-product-compliance
Lightning Source LLC
Chambersburg PA
CBHW061558250726
48657CB00021B/2283